The Fastest G

Mediterranean Diet

Super-Quick and Easy Recipes to Boost Your Diet and Save Your Time

Raphael Chapman

Table of contents

4

Mediterranean Fish and Pasta Stew

Preparation Time: 20 minutes

Cooking Time: 30 minutes

Servings: 4

Ingredients:

- Onions – 2 (chopped)
- Crushed tomatoes – 1 (28 oz.) can
- Fresh parsley – ½ cup (chopped)
- Worcestershire sauce – 2 tbsp.
- Paprika – 1 tsp.
- Dry pasta – 3 oz.
- Garlic – 4 cloves (minced)
- Olive oil – 1 tbsp.
- Water – 6 cups
- Fresh cilantro – ½ cup (chopped)
- Ground cinnamon – 1 tsp.
- Cod fillets – 1 ½ lb. (cubed)
- Salt to taste
- Ground black pepper – 1 tbsp.

Directions:

1. In a large pot, sauté the onions and garlic in the olive oil for 5 minutes over medium heat while stirring constantly.
2. Add tomatoes with the liquid, parsley, water and cilantro. Bring the mixture to boil and reduce heat to low and simmer for about 15 minutes.

3. Stir in the Worcestershire sauce, paprika, cinnamon and fish, the simmer over medium heat for 10 minutes. Add the pasta and simmer for about 8 minutes more or until the pasta is tender.

4. Season with salt and ground pepper to taste.

Nutrition: Calories: 237; Fat: 4.2 g; Carbs: 26.2 g; Protein: 25.3 g;

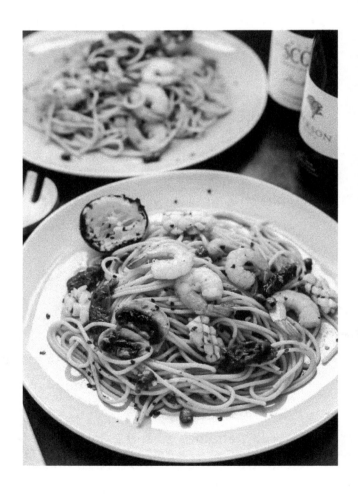

Parsley Pesto Paste

Preparation Time: 5 minutes

Cooking Time: 15 minutes

Servings: 4

Ingredients:

- 2 cups of parsley leaves
- 1/2 cup of grated parmesan cheese
- Two cloves of garlic
- 1/2 cup lemon juice
- 1/4 cup olive oil
- 1/3 cup pine nut
- Table salt to taste

Directions:

1. Put all ingredients except the parmesan cheese in a food processor then pulse until smooth.
2. Remove from the blender, add grated parmesan and gently stir.
3. Serve.

Nutrition: Calories 266, Fat 25g, Carbs 6g, Protein 8g

Potato in Tomato Paste

Preparation Time: 25 minutes

Cooking Time: 30 minutes

Servings: 4

Ingredients:

- Four large cubed potatoes
- 1 Tbsp aromatic dry spices mix
- One onion, chopped
- 4 Tbsp Olive oil
- Black pepper
- One minced garlic clove
- 1 cup tomato paste
- 1 cup of water
- Chopped parsley,
- Salt

Directions:

1. Heat the olive oil in a pan over medium heat and sauté the onion until translucent.
2. Add the potatoes, the spice mixture and continue to sauté.
3. Add the garlic, tomato paste, diced tomato, water, salt and pepper, and stir.
4. Cover the pot and cook for half an hour over low heat.
5. Serve with fresh coriander.

Nutrition: Calories 312, Fat 14g, Carbs 43g, Protein 6g

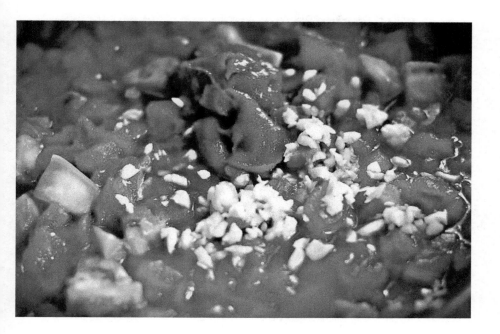

Hummus

Preparation Time: 15 minutes

Cooking Time: 10 minutes

Servings: 4

Ingredients:

- 1/2 cup tahini
- 1 tsp salt
- Two cloves garlic halved
- 1 tbsp olive oil
- 2 cup canned garbanzo beans, drained
- 1/2 cup lemon juice
- 1 tbsp paprika
- 1 tsp parsley

Directions:

1. Pulse the garlic, lemon juice, garbanzos, salt, and tahini in a food processor until smooth.
2. Add this to a bowl with olive oil, paprika, and parsley.
3. Enjoy.

Nutrition: Calories 77 Fat 4.3 g Carbs 8.1g Protein 2.6 g

Hollandaise Sauce

Preparation Time: 10 minutes

Cooking Time: 5 minutes

Servings: 1

Ingredients:

- One lemon (Zested and juiced)
- One tsp garlic powder
- 1/2 tsp cayenne pepper
- 1/2 cup cashew butter
- Two tsp Dijon mustard
- 1/2 cup of warm water
- 1/2 tsp ground turmeric

Directions:

1. In a food processor, put all ingredients, and then pulse until smooth.
2. Put it in a sealed container and refrigerate it for up to three days.
3. Enjoy.

Nutrition: Calories 150 Protein 6 g Fat 12 g Carbs 10 g

Creamy Tahini Dip

Preparation Time: 5 minutes

Cooking Time: 4 minutes

Servings: 4

Ingredients:

- Half a lemon (Juiced)
- One crushed garlic clove
- Salt
- 1/2 cup tahini
- 2 cups of water
- Fresh parsley, chopped
- Black pepper

Directions:

1. Put the tahini, salt, lemon juice, garlic, and a little water in a bowl then stir until the tahini becomes white and smooth.
2. Sprinkle the parsley and black pepper and serve.
3. Enjoy.

Nutrition: Calories 93 Protein 2.6 g Fat 8.1 g Carbs 4.4 g

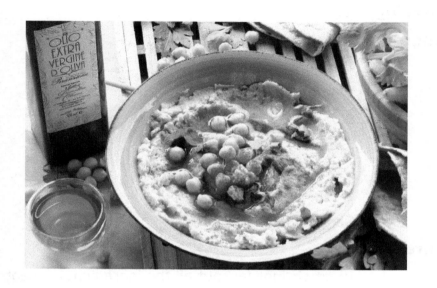

Basil Lime Dip

Preparation Time: 5 minutes

Cooking Time: 10 minutes

Servings: 16

Ingredients:

- Ten garlic cloves, crushed
- 1/4 cup brown rice syrup
- 8 oz. hemp oil
- One tsp of sea salt
- One pinch xanthan gum
- 1 1/2 cups chopped basil,
- Six tbsp key lime juice

Directions:

1. In an airtight jar, put all the ingredients except the xanthan gum, and then shake to well.
2. Put the mixture plus the xanthan, into a blender and pulse.
3. Return the mixture in the jar.
4. Enjoy.

Nutrition: Calories 143 Cholesterol 0 mg Fat 14 g Carbs 6 g

Cilantro Dip

Preparation Time: 5 minutes

Cooking Time: 4 minutes

Servings: 7

Ingredients:

- 12 cloves of garlic
- 4 cups cilantro leaves
- One tsp salt
- 1/2 tsp ground black pepper
- 1 cup olive oil

Directions:

1. Add all ingredients to a blender and pulse until velvety.
2. You can put in the refrigerator for up to two days.
3. Enjoy.

Nutrition: Calories 230; Fat 20.5 g; Carbs 7.1 g; Protein 5 g

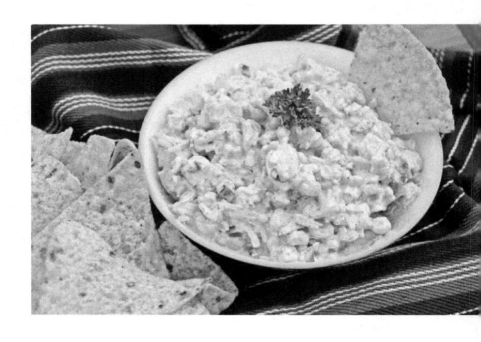

Tahini Sauce

Preparation Time: 7 minutes

Cooking Time: 5 minutes

Servings: 6

Ingredients:

- Four mashed garlic cloves
- Salt to taste
- 1 cup tahini paste
- 1/2 cup lemon juice
- Seven tbsp water

Directions:

1. Put all ingredients in a bowl and whisk until well combined.
2. Refrigerate up to 5 days.
3. Enjoy.

Nutrition: Calories 77; Fat 6.6 g; Carbs 3.2 g; Protein 2.3 g

Arugula Salsa

Preparation Time: 5 minutes

Cooking Time: 20 minutes

Servings: 6

Ingredients:

- 30 Kalamata olives, pitted, quartered
- Three tbsp olive oil
- One chopped red bell pepper
- One chopped yellow bell pepper
- Two tsp fennel seeds, crushed
- 1 cup baby arugula, chopped

Directions:

1. Heat oil in a pan over medium heat.
2. Add fennel seeds and sauté until fragrant.
3. Add bell peppers and sauté until they are soft.
4. Transfer into a bowl.
5. Add salt, pepper, and arugula and stir until arugula wilts.
6. Enjoy.

Nutrition: Calories 16; Fat 0.1 g; Carbs 3.9 g; Protein 0.6 g

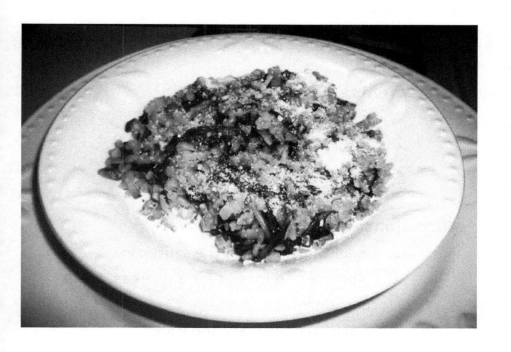

Fragrant Basmati Rice

Preparation Time: 5 minutes

Cooking Time: 17 minutes

Servings: 6

Ingredients:

- 1 cup long-grain rice
- 1 tbsp. olive oil
- 1 tsp. dried rosemary
- 2 ½ cup water

Directions:

1. Heat the olive oil in the saucepan.
2. Add rice and roast it for 2 minutes. Stir it constantly.
3. Then add rosemary and water.
4. Stir the rice and close the lid.
5. Cook it for 15 minutes or until it soaks all water.

Nutrition:

Calories: 334;

Protein: 12.3g;

Carbs: 19.4g;

Fat: 6.3g

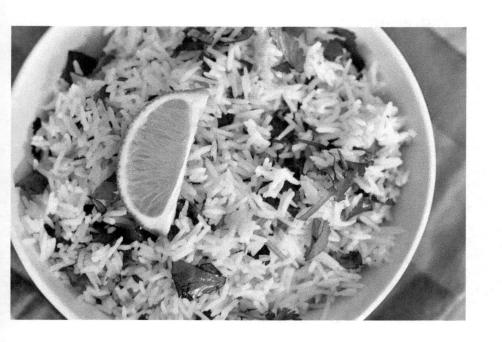

Cranberry Rice

Preparation Time: 5 minutes

Cooking Time: 20 minutes

Servings: 4

Ingredients:

- ¼ cup basmati rice
- 1 cup of organic almond milk
- 2 oz dried cranberries
- ¼ tsp. ground cinnamon

Directions:

1. Put all ingredients in the saucepan, stir, and close the lid.
2. Cook the rice on low heat for 20 minutes.

Nutrition:

Calories: 153;

Protein: 12.3g;

Carbs: 3.4g;

Fat: 6.3g

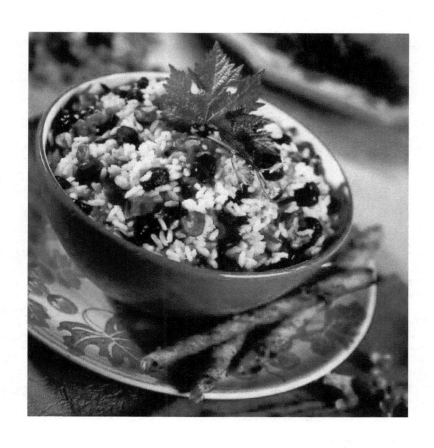

Italian Style Wild Rice

Preparation Time: minutes

Cooking Time: 20 minutes

Servings: 6

Ingredients:

- 1 cup wild rice
- 3 cups chicken stock
- 1 tsp. Italian seasonings
- 2 oz Feta, crumbled
- 1 tbsp. olive oil

Directions:

1. Mix wild rice with olive oil and chicken stock.
2. Close the lid and cook it for 25 minutes over the medium-low heat.
3. Then add Italian seasonings and crumbled feta.
4. Stir the rice.

Nutrition:

Calories: 253;

Protein: 15.3g;

Carbs: 3.4g;

Fat: 6.3g

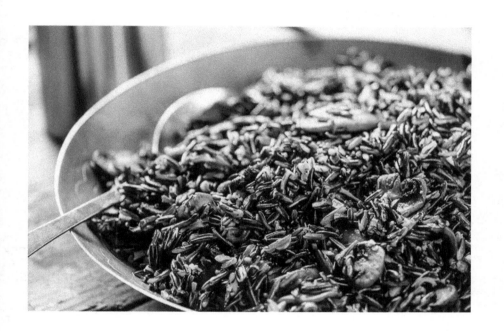

Brown Rice Saute

Preparation Time: 5 minutes

Cooking Time: 20 minutes

Servings: 3

Ingredients:

- 3 oz brown rice
- 9 oz chicken stock
- 1 tsp. curry powder
- 1 onion, diced
- 4 tbsp. olive oil

Directions:

1. Heat olive oil in the saucepan.
2. Add onion and cook it until light brown.
3. Add brown rice, curry powder, and chicken stock.
4. Close the lid and saute the rice for 15 minutes.

Nutrition:

Calories: 237;

Protein: 12.3g;

Carbs: 3.4g;

Fat: 6.3g

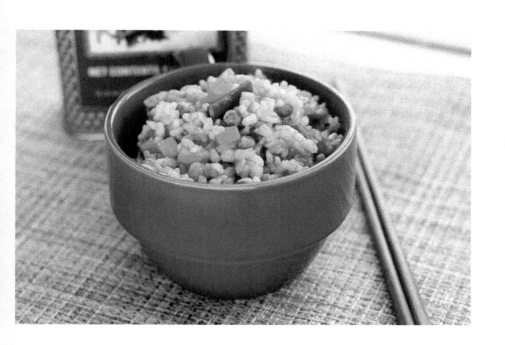

Pesto Rice

Preparation Time: 8 minutes

Cooking Time: 15 minutes

Servings: 4

Ingredients:

- ½ cup of basmati rice
- 1.5cup of water
- 2 tbsp. pesto sauce

Directions:

1. Simmer the rice water for 15 minutes on the low heat or until the rice soaks all liquid.
2. Then mix cooked tice with pesto sauce.

Nutrition:

Calories: 353;

Protein: 12.3g;

Carbs: 3.4g;

Fat: 6.3g

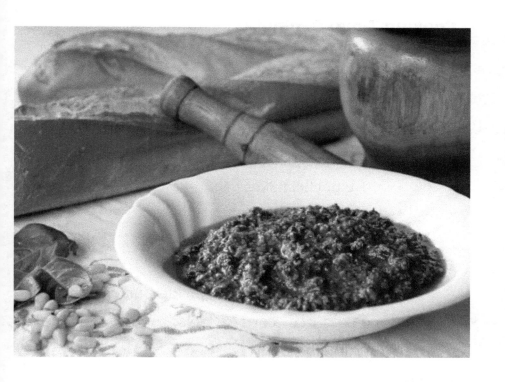

Rice Salad

Preparation Time: 10 minutes

Cooking Time: 0 minutes

Servings: 4

Ingredients:

- ½ cup long-grain rice, cooked
- ½ cup corn kernels, cooked
- 1 tomato, chopped
- 1 tsp. chili flakes
- ¼ cup plain yogurt
- 1 cucumber pickle

Directions:

1. Grate the cucumber pickle and mix it with cooked rice, corn kernels, tomato, chili flakes, and plain yogurt.

Nutrition:

Calories: 153;

Protein: 12.3g;

Carbs: 18.4g;

Fat: 6.3g

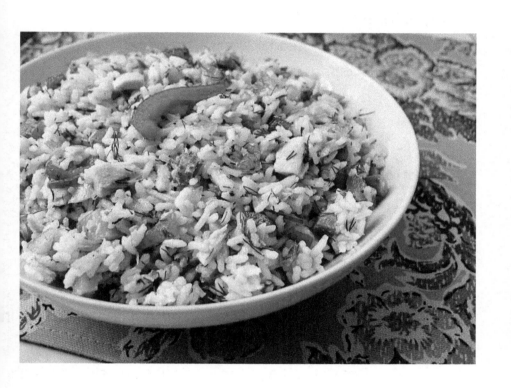

Rice Meatballs

Preparation Time: 10 minutes

Cooking Time: 15 minutes

Servings: 20

Ingredients:

- ¼ cup Cheddar cheese, shredded
- 1 tsp. ground black pepper
- 1 cup of basmati rice, cooked
- ¼ cup ground chicken
- 1 tsp. olive oil

Directions:

1. In the mixing bowl, mix Cheddar cheese, ground black pepper, rice, and ground chicken.
2. Then make the balls from the mixture.
3. Heat the olive oil well and put the rice balls in the hot oil.
4. Roast the balls for 1 minute per side on high heat.
5. Then transfer the balls in the oven and bake them for 20 minutes at 360F.

Nutrition:

Calories: 183;

Protein: 12.3g;

Carbs:17g

Fat: 6.3g

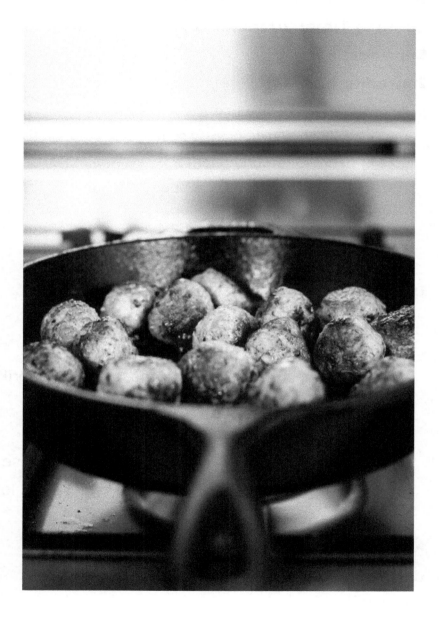

Mediterranean Paella

Preparation Time: 10 minutes

Cooking Time: 30 minutes

Servings: 6

Ingredients:

- 1 cup risotto rice
- 2 oz yellow onion, diced
- ½ tsp. ground paprika
- 1 cup tomatoes, chopped
- 1 cup shrimps, peeled
- 1 tsp. olive oil
- 3 cups of water

Directions:

1. Heat olive oil in the saucepan.
2. Add onion and cook it for 2 minutes.
3. Then stir well, add shrimps, ground paprika, tomatoes, and stir well.
4. Cook the ingredients for 5 minutes.
5. Add water and risotto rice. Stir well, close the lid, and cook the meal for 20 minutes on low heat.

Nutrition:

Calories: 223;

Carbs:21g;

Protein: 12.3g;

Fat: 6.3g

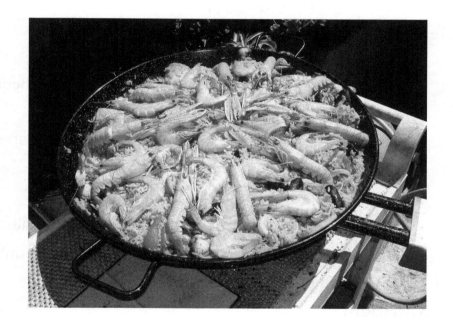

Fast Chicken Rice

Preparation Time: 10 minutes

Cooking Time: 20 minutes

Servings: 5

Ingredients:

- 1 cup basmati rice
- 3 tbsp. avocado oil
- 2.5cups chicken stock
- ½ tsp. dried dill
- 10 oz chicken breast, skinless, boneless, chopped

Directions:

1. Mix oil with rice and roast it in the saucepan for 5 minutes over the low heat.
2. Then add chicken and chicken stock.
3. Add dill, stir the ingredients and cook the meal on medium heat for 15 minutes or until all ingredients are cooked.

Nutrition:

Calories: 213;

Protein: 12.3g;

Carbs:14g

Fat: 6.3g

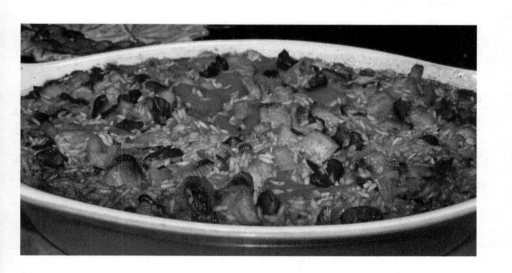

Rice Jambalaya

Preparation Time: 5 minutes

Cooking Time: 30 minutes

Servings: 8

Ingredients:

- 1 cup tomatoes, chopped
- 1 cup bell pepper, chopped
- ¼ cup carrot, chopped
- 1 tsp. cayenne pepper
- 4 cups chicken stock
- 1 cup of basmati rice
- 2 tbsp. olive oil
- ½ cup chickpeas, cooked

Directions:

1. Melt the olive oil and add carrot, bell pepper, and tomatoes.
2. Cook the vegetables for 10 minutes on medium heat.
3. Then add chicken stock, chickpeas, and rice.

4. Add cayenne pepper and stir the meal.

5. Close the lid and cook it for 20 minutes on low heat.

Nutrition:

Calories: 263;

Protein: 10.3g;

Carbs: 3.4g;

Fat: 6.3g

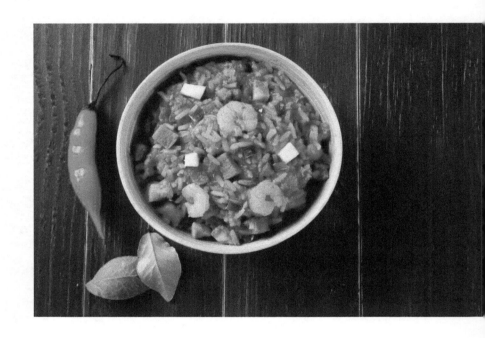

Jasmine Rice with Scallions

Preparation Time: 10 minutes

Cooking Time: 10 minutes

Servings: 6

Ingredients:

- 3 tbsp. olive oil
- 1 cup jasmine rice
- 2 tbsp. scallions, chopped
- ½ tsp. ground black pepper
- 2 tsp. lemon juice

Directions:

1. Cook the rice according to the directions of the manufacturer.
2. Then add scallions, olive oil, ground black pepper, and lemon juice.
3. Carefully stir the meal.

Nutrition:

Calories: 189;

Protein: 12.3g;

Carbs:17g

Fat: 6.3g

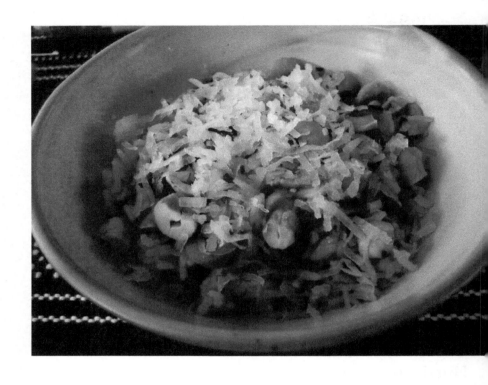

Cremini Mushrooms Pilaf

Preparation Time: 10 minutes

Cooking Time: 25 minutes

Servings: 6

Ingredients:

- 2 cups of water
- ½ cup white onion, diced
- 1 cup cremini mushrooms, chopped
- 1 cup of basmati rice
- ¼ tsp. lime zest, grated
- 2 oz goat cheese, crumbled
- 2 tbsp. olive oil

Directions:

1. Put rice in the saucepan.
2. Add water and cook for 15 minutes over the low heat.
3. Then roast the mushrooms with olive oil, lime zest, and white onion in the skillet until they are light brown.
4. Add the cooked mushrooms in the cooked rice. Stir well.
5. Top the meal with crumbled goat cheese.

Nutrition:

Calories: 193;

Protein: 12.3g;

Carbs:18g

Fat: 6.3g

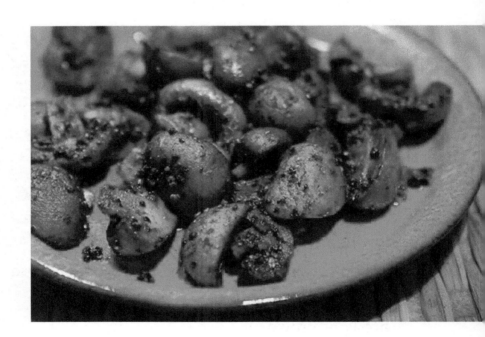

Vegetable Rice

Preparation Time: 10 minutes

Cooking Time: 30 minutes

Servings: 6

Ingredients:

- 2 cups wild rice
- 1 tsp. Italian seasonings
- 1 tbsp. olive oil
- ¼ cup carrot, diced
- ½ cup snap peas, frozen
- 5 cups of water

Directions:

1. Mix 4 cups of water and wild rice in the saucepan.
2. Cook the rice for 15 minutes or until the rice soaks all liquid.
3. Then heat the olive oil in the separated saucepan.
4. Add carrot and roast it until light brown.
5. Add snap peas, water, and rice.
6. Stir well and close the lid.
7. Cook the rice for 10 minutes.

Nutrition:

Calories: 187;

Protein: 12.3g;

Carbs:14g

Fat: 4.3g

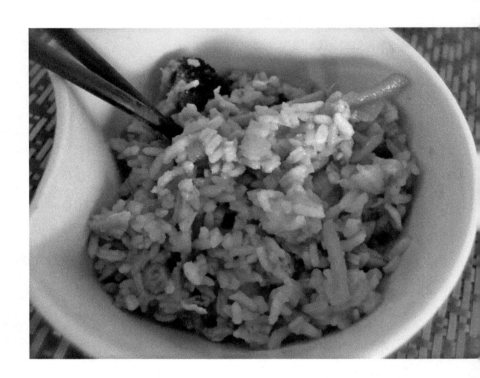

Tomato Rice

Preparation Time: 10 minutes

Cooking Time: 20 minutes

Servings: 4

Ingredients:

- 1 cup basmati rice
- 3 cups chicken stock
- 1 tsp. ground coriander
- ¼ tsp. dried thyme
- 2 tbsp. olive oil
- 2 tbsp. tomato paste

Directions:

1. Roast the rice with olive oil in the saucepan for 5 minutes. Stir it.
2. Then add thyme, coriander, and tomato paste.
3. Add water, mix the rice mixture, and close the lid.
4. Cook the rice for 15 minutes over the medium heat.

Nutrition:

Calories: 53;

Protein: 12.3g;

Carbs: 13g;

Fat: 6.3g

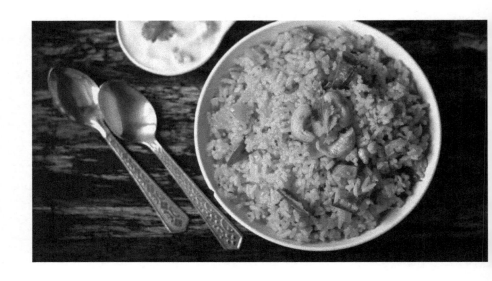

Rice with Grilled Tomatoes

Preparation Time: 10 minutes

Cooking Time: 20 minutes

Servings: 6

Ingredients:

- 1 cup of basmati rice
- cups chicken stock
- 1 tsp. olive oil
- 2 tomatoes, roughly sliced

Directions:

1. Sprinkle the tomatoes with olive oil and grill in the preheated to 400F grill for 1 minute per side.
2. Then cook rice with chicken stock for 15 minutes.
3. Transfer the cooked rice in the bowls and top with grilled tomatoes.

Nutrition:

Calories: 83;

Protein: 12.3g;

Carbs: 13g

Fat: 6.3g

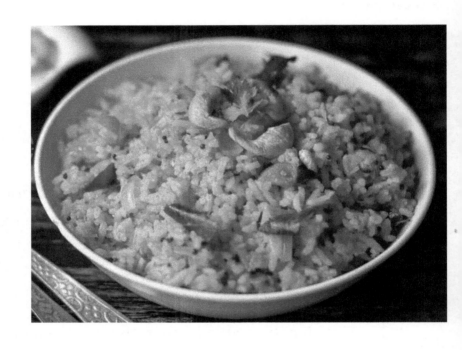

Rice and Meat Salad

Preparation Time: 10 minutes

Cooking Time: 0 minutes

Servings: 6

Ingredients:

- 1 cup white cabbage, shredded
- 1 cup long grain rice, cooked
- 8 oz beef steak, cooked, cut into the strips
- 1/3 cup plain yogurt
- 1 tsp. salt
- 1 tsp. chives, chopped

Directions:

1. Put cabbage and rice in the big bowl.
2. Add white rice and meat strips.
3. Then add plain yogurt, chives, and salt.
4. Stir the salad until homogenous.

Nutrition:

Calories: 123;

Protein: 14.3g;

Carbs: 12.8g;

Fat: 6.3g

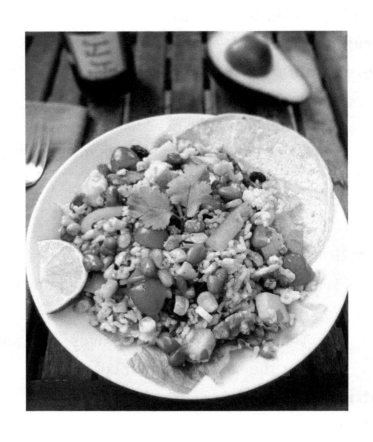

Rice Bowl

Preparation Time: 10 minutes

Cooking Time: 0 minutes

Servings: 6

Ingredients:

- 1 cup of basmati rice, cooked
- 4 oz beef sirloin, grilled
- ½ cup tomatoes, chopped
- 2 tbsp. soy sauce
- 1 tsp. ground paprika
- 2 oz scallions, sliced

Directions:

1. Put the cooked rice in the serving bowls.
2. Add beef sirloin, tomatoes, and scallions.
3. Then sprinkle the meal with soy sauce and ground paprika.

Nutrition:

Calories: 63;

Protein: 12.3g;

Carbs: 13.7g;

Fat: 6.3g

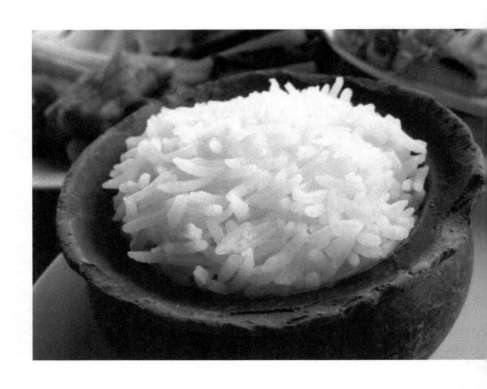

Zucchini Rice

Preparation Time: 10 minutes

Cooking Time: 25 minutes

Servings: 2

Ingredients:

- ½ cup of long grain rice
- 1 cup chicken stock
- 1 zucchini, cubed
- 1 tbsp. olive oil
- 1 tsp. curry powder
- 1 tbsp. raisins

Directions:

1. Mix rice and chicken stock in the saucepan and cook for 15 minutes or until the rice soaks the liquid.
2. Then heat the olive oil.
3. Add zucchini in the oil and roast for 5 minutes.
4. After this, sprinkle the zucchini with curry powder, add raisins and rice.
5. Carefully mix the rice and cook for 5 minutes.

Nutrition:

Calories: 113;

Protein: 12.3g;

Carbs: 14g;

Fat: 4.3g

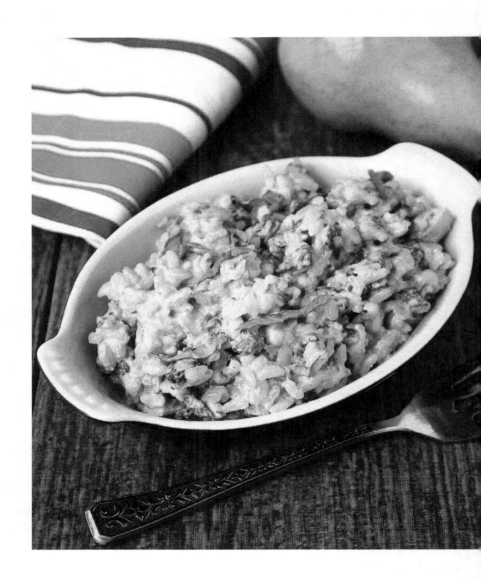

Rice Soup

Preparation Time: 10 minutes

Cooking Time: 20 minutes

Servings: 4

Ingredients:

- 3 cups chicken stock
- ½ lb. chicken breast, shredded
- 1 tbsp. chives, chopped
- 1 egg, whisked
- ½ white onion, diced
- 1 bell pepper, chopped
- 1 tbsp. olive oil
- ¼ cup arborio rice
- ½ tsp. salt
- 1 tbsp. fresh cilantro, chopped

Directions:

1. Pour olive oil in the stock pan and preheat it.

2. Add onion and bell pepper. Roast the vegetables for 3-4 minutes. Stir them from time to time.
3. After this, add rice and stir well.
4. Cook the ingredients for 3 minutes over the medium heat.
5. Then add chicken stock and stir the soup well.
6. Add salt and bring the soup to boil.
7. Add shredded chicken breast, cilantro, and chives. Add egg and stir it carefully.
8. Close the lid and simmer the soup for 5 minutes over the medium heat.
9. Remove the cooked soup from the heat.

Nutrition:

Calories 176,

Fat 7.6g,

Carbs: 9g

Protein 15.2g

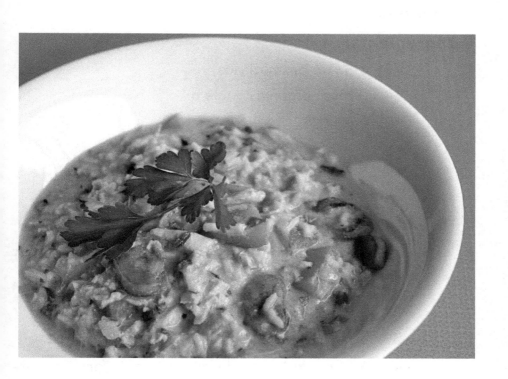

Rice with Prunes

Preparation Time: 5 minutes

Cooking Time: 20 minutes

Servings: 7

Ingredients:

- 1.5 cup basmati rice
- 3 tbsp. organic canola oil
- 5 prunes, chopped
- ¼ cup cream cheese
- 3.5 cups water
- ½ tsp. salt

Directions:

1. Mix water and basmati rice in the saucepan and boil for 15 minutes on low heat.
2. Then add cream cheese, salt, and prunes.
3. Stir the rice carefully and bring it to boil.
4. Add organic canola oil and cook for 1 minute more.

Nutrition:

Calories: 83;

Protein: 12.3g;

Carbs: 12g;

Fat: 6.3g

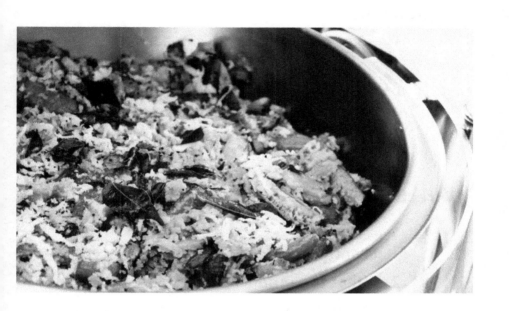

Rice and Fish Cakes

Preparation Time: 10 minutes

Cooking Time: 10 minutes

Servings: 6

Ingredients:

- 6 oz salmon, canned, shredded
- 1 egg, beaten
- ¼ cup of basmati rice, cooked
- 1 tsp. dried cilantro
- ½ tsp. chili flakes
- 1 tbsp. organic canola oil

Directions:

1. Mix salmon with egg, basmati rice, dried cilantro, and chili flakes.
2. Heat the organic canola oil in the skillet.
3. Make the small cakes from the salmon mixture and put in the hot oil.
4. Roast the cakes for 2 minutes per side or until they are light brown.

Nutrition:

Calories: 123;

Protein: 12.3g;

Carbs: 7g;

Fat: 6.3g

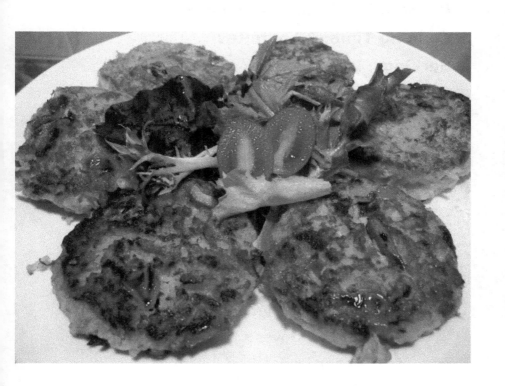

Carbonara Pasta With Champignons

Preparation Time: 10 minutes

Cooking Time: 25 minutes

Servings: 2

Ingredients :

- Spaghetti 9 oz.
- Bacon 7 oz.
- Cream 20% 7 oz.
- Parmesan Cheese 3.5 oz.
- Egg yolk 4 pieces
- Garlic 5 cloves
- Champignons 5 oz.
- Olive oil 10 ml
- Salt to taste
- Ground black pepper to taste

Directions:

1. Prepare the ingredients.

2. Cut the bacon into strips, chop the garlic finely, chop the mushrooms.
3. Fry the garlic in a pan, then the mushrooms and bacon.
4. Grate the parmesan.
5. Put egg yolks in a plate, salt, pepper and beat.
6. Add cream and grated cheese to the yolks, mix.
7. Boil spaghetti to al dente (about a minute less than indicated on the packet).
8. Put the spaghetti in a pan, add the sauce, bacon and mushrooms.

Nutrition:

Calories: 767

Protein: 18 g

Fat: 32 g

Carbs: 33 g

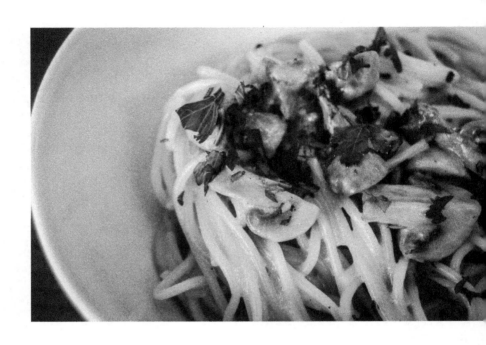

Spaghetti Carbonara With Red Onion

Preparation Time: 15 minutes

Cooking Time: 25 minutes

Servings: 4

Ingredients :

- Spaghetti 9 oz.
- Butter 3/4 oz.
- Garlic 2 cloves
- Red onion 1 head
- Bacon 2 oz.
- Cream 20% 200 ml
- Grated Parmesan Cheese 2 oz.
- 4 eggs
- Saltto taste
- Ground black pepper to taste

Directions:

1. Boil water in a large saucepan and cook the pasta until al dente. Usually for this you need to

cook it for a minute less than indicated on the pack.

2.   While the pasta is boiling, melt the butter in a pan and fry finely chopped onion, garlic and bacon on it. To softness and to a distinct garlic and fried bacon smell.

3.   Remove the pan from the heat and beat four egg yolks with cream and grated Parmesan in a deep bowl. Salt and pepper the mixture, whisk again.

4.   In the prepared spaghetti, pour the pieces of bacon fried with onions and garlic. Pour in a mixture of cream, yolks and parmesan, mix. And serve immediately, sprinkled with freshly grated cheese and black pepper

Nutrition:

Calories: 307

Protein: 18 g

Fat: 14 g

Carbs: 33 g

Cuttlefish Pasta With Carbonara Sauce

Preparation Time: 15 minutes

Cooking Time: 30 minutes

Servings: 3

Ingredients :

- Pasta 7 oz.
- Smoked bacon 5 oz.
- Grated Parmesan Cheese 2 oz.
- Champignons 7 oz.
- Cream 200 ml
- Egg yolk 1 piece
- Garlic 3 cloves
- Butter 2 tbsp.
- Ground black pepper pinch
- Ground nutmeg pinch

Directions:

1. Boil spaghetti. At this time, fry the garlic and bacon in butter for three minutes.

2.   Add the mushroom slices to the bacon, mix and fry for eight to ten minutes. During this time, the spaghetti will cook, drain from them and add to the mushrooms and bacon.

3.   The final stage - cream, egg yolk, ground black pepper, ground nutmeg and grated cheese. Beat all this and pour spaghetti, fry for five minutes and serve.

Nutrition:

Calories: 593

Protein: 18 g

Fat: 14 g

Carbs: 33 g

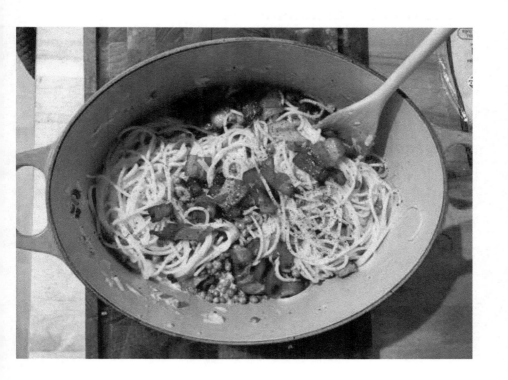

Spaghetti Carbonara

Preparation Time: 10 minutes

Cooking Time: 25 minutes

Servings: 2

Ingredients:

- Spaghetti 160 g
- Pancetta 4 oz.
- Hard cheese 2 oz.
- Egg yolk 2 pieces
- Salt to taste
- Freshly ground black pepper to taste

Directions:

1. Bring well-salted water to a boil. Cook spaghetti to al dente. Save a little broth from the paste; you may need it. Drain the rest.
2. While preparing the pasta, heat the pan and fry the pancetta on it until golden, remove from heat.

3. In a small bowl, beat the yolks with grated cheese until smooth.

4. Return the pan with the pancetta to a small fire, add about 50 ml of the broth from the pasta, throw the spaghetti there and mix well until the boiling stops. Most of the water should boil.

5. Remove the pan from the heat and add the yolks with cheese and mix quickly until the yolks thicken. If the sauce seems too thick, add a little more paste broth. Pepper and salt to taste, serve.

Nutrition:

Calories: 702

Protein: 18 g

Fat: 14 g

Carbs: 33 g

Chanterelle Pasta

Preparation Time: 15 minutes

Cooking Time: 30 minutes

Servings: 4

Ingredients:

- Chanterelles 7 oz.
- Tagliatelle pasta 7 oz.
- Tomato Sauce 7 oz.
- Garlic 2 cloves
- Olive oil 20 ml
- Dry white wine 30 ml
- Butter 10 g
- Parmesan Cheese 2 oz.
- Saltto taste
- Ground black pepper to taste

Directions:

1. Heat olive oil in a pan with a thick bottom, add a couple of whole cloves of garlic, add chanterelles (pre-washed and well-dried).
2. Fry the chanterelles 5-7 minutes until golden brown, pour in white wine, evaporate.
3. Then pour the tomato sauce and simmer for about 5 minutes. At the end, add butter, salt and pepper.
4. Add the paste cooked al-dente to the sauce and mix. Serve garnished with sliced parmesan and parsley.

Nutrition:

Calories: 360

Protein: 18 g

Fat: 16 g

Carbs: 32 g

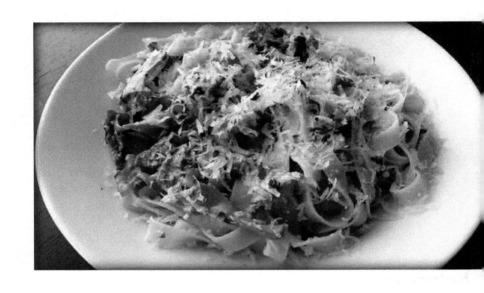

Pasta "Verochka"

Preparation Time: 5 minutes

Cooking Time: 20 minutes

Servings: 2

Ingredients:

- Spaghetti 10 oz.
- Cream 33% 200 ml
- Lightly salted trout 3.5 oz.
- Grated Parmesan Cheese 2 oz.
- Dried oregano to taste
- Dried basil to taste

Directions:

1. Boil spaghetti - or other suitable pasta - until cooked, following the time indicated on the package. You do not need to salt water - the salt will give the fish.

2. Meanwhile, finely chop the red fish - not necessarily trout, any. And its quantity may be different - if only the fish had no more pasta.

3. Heat the cream in a pan (it is better to take Fatter) and add fish to them. Keep on fire, stirring constantly and, most importantly, not boiling. When the fish loses color, you can remove the pan from the heat.
4. Throw the prepared pasta into a colander and add to the sauce. Or add the sauce to the paste - as anyone is more familiar and convenient. Add oregano and basil, mix.
5. Sprinkle the paste spread on the plates with grated Parmesan.

Nutrition:

Calories: 687

Protein: 18 g

Fat: 14 g

Carbs: 33 g

Pasta e Patate

Preparation Time: 15 minutes

Cooking Time: 30 minutes

Servings: 3

Ingredients:

- Bacon 5 oz.
- Onions 3 oz.
- Spaghetti 8 oz.
- Potato14 oz.
- Parmesan Cheese 3 oz.
- Olive oil 30 ml
- Freshly ground black pepper to taste
- Salt to taste

Directions:

1. Fry the bacon in a dry skillet. Add olive oil and fry finely chopped onions, not until golden brown.

2. Add chopped potatoes to the onion, fry and add water to the onion. Cook until al dente, 5-10 minutes.

3. Break the spaghetti, toss it to the potatoes, add water, continue cooking until the spaghetti is ready. Pour a little water over the entire cooking process so that a little liquid is left in the finale, sufficient to make a sauce.

4. In the finale add grated parmesan, olive oil, freshly ground black pepper, mix well

Nutrition:

Calories: 615

Protein: 18 g

Fat: 29 g

Carbs: 33 g

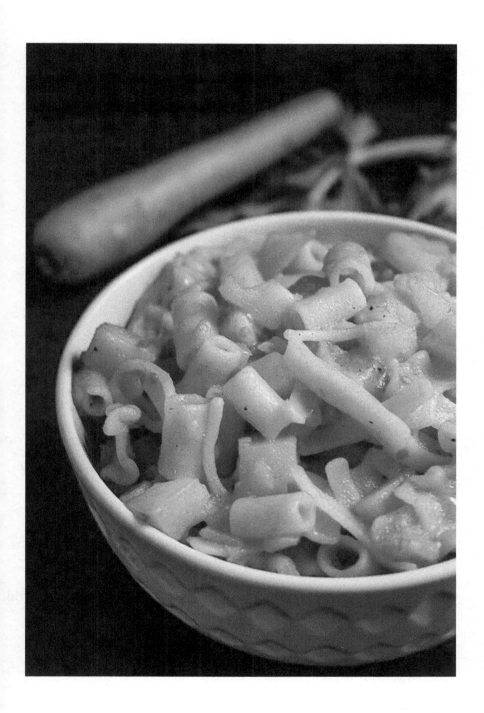

Pasta with Fresh Tomatoes

Preparation Time: 15 minutes

Cooking Time: 30 minutes

Servings: 3

Ingredients:

- Tagliatelle pasta 7 oz.
- Tomatoes 1 piece
- 5 black olives
- Garlic 2 cloves
- Olive oil 50 ml

Directions:

1. Boil the pasta in salted boiling water.
2. Simultaneously in 1 tbsp. of olive oil, lightly fry the garlic and sliced olives.
3. Dice the fresh tomatoes and add to the garlic an olives. Cooking tomatoes is not necessary, they should only warm up.
4. Slightly salt and pepper the sauce.
5. Drain the water and combine the pasta with the sauce.
6. Put the pasta in a plate and lightly pour olive oil.

Nutrition:

Calories: 667

Protein: 18 g

Fat: 52 g

Carbs: 33 g

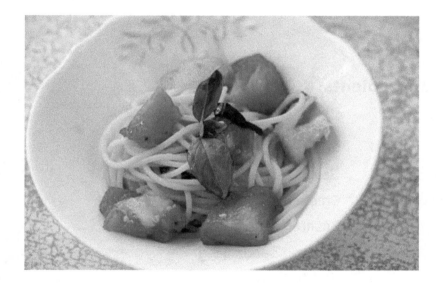

Spaghetti Carbonara With Chicken

Preparation Time: 5 minutes

Cooking Time: 30 minutes

Servings: 2

Ingredients:

- Durum wheat spaghetti 10 oz.
- Cream 100 ml
- Garlic 2 cloves
- Chicken egg 3 pieces
- Basilto taste
- Sesame seeds 15 g
- Saltto taste
- Olive oil 3 tbsp.
- Parmesan Cheese 2 oz.
- Chicken fillet 7 oz.

Directions:

1. Finely chop the chicken fillet and fry in olive oil until tender.

2.   Peel the garlic, chop finely and add to the chicken. Fry it all together for 1-2 minutes. Then add cream, salt to taste. Stew on low heat so that the cream does not curl.
3.   Add a spoonful of olive oil to boiling water, salt to taste to taste. Cooking spaghetti to al dente.
4.   Cooking the sauce. To do this, beat the eggs, then add basil, salt, sesame and grated parmesan.
5.   Once the spaghetti is ready, we discard them in a colander, then - in a pan with chicken and garlic, pour everything in the resulting sauce and simmer for another 2-3 minutes over low heat.

Nutrition:

Calories: 624

Protein: 18 g

Fat: 28 g

Carbs: 33 g

Carbonara With Fettuccine

Preparation Time: 10 minutes

Cooking Time: 25 minutes

Servings: 4

Ingredients:

- Fettuccine Pasta 17 oz.
- Bacon 8 slices
- 4 eggs
- Grated Parmesan Cheese 2 oz.
- Cream 315 ml

Directions:

1. Cut the bacon into thin strips and fry in a pan over medium heat until crisp. Lay on a paper towel.
2. Put the pasta in a pot of boiling salted water and cook until cooked. Drain and return to pan.
3. While the pasta is boiling, beat the eggs with cream and parmesan until smooth. Add the bacon

and mix well. Pour the sauce into a hot paste and mix well.

4.   Return to a frying pan to a very small fire and simmer a little less than 1 minute until the sauce thickens slightly.

Nutrition:

Calories: 916

Protein: 18 g

Fat: 41 g

Carbs: 33 g

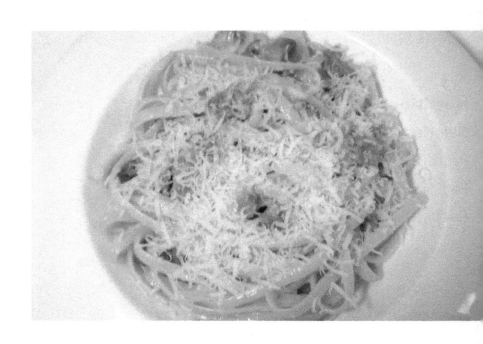

Fast Spaghetti Carbonara
Preparation Time: 5 minutes

Cooking Time: 30 minutes

Servings: 3

Ingredients:

- Spaghetti 3 oz.
- Bacon 1.5 oz.
- Cream 35% 50 ml
- Chicken egg 1 piece
- Dry white wine 20 ml
- Grana padano cheese 0.8 oz.

Directions:

1. We put spaghetti in boiling water, cook for 12 minutes, put it in a sieve.
2. At the chicken egg, we separate the yolk from the Protein, mix the yolks with animal cream, grana padano cheese, and pepper.
3. Cut the bacon with a large plate into large plates, fry in butter, add dry white wine and olive oil.
4. Into the fried bacon with wine and oil we introduce ready-made spaghetti, add the mass with egg and cream, mix quickly

Nutrition:

Calories: 847

Protein: 18 g

Fat: 49 g

Carbs: 33 g

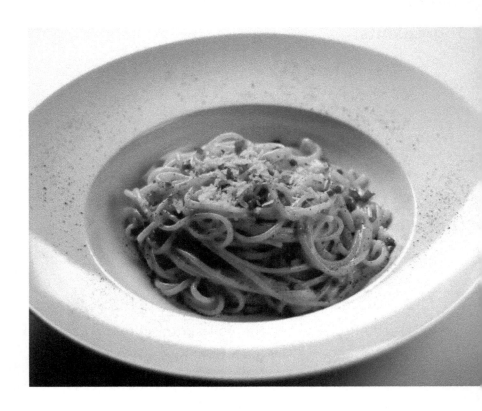

Pasta with Greens

Preparation Time: 35 Minutes
 Servings: 8

Ingredients:

- Swiss chard – 1 bunch (remove the stems)
- Oil packed sun-dried tomatoes – ½ cup (chopped)
- Green olives – ½ cup (chopped and pitted)
- Fresh parmesan cheese – ¼ cup (grated)
- Dry fusilli pasta – 1 (16 oz.) package
- Olive oil – 2 tbsp.
- Kalamata olives – ½ cup (chopped and pitted)
- Garlic – 1 clove (minced)

Directions:

1. Cook pasta in lightly salted water for 10 to 12 minutes until al dente then drain.
2. Put the chard in a microwave safe bowl, fill with water until it is about ½ filled with water. Cook on high in the microwave for about 5 minutes until the chard is limp then drain.

3. Over medium heat, heat the oil in a skillet. Stir in the oil, the sun-dried tomatoes, green olives, kalamata olives and garlic.
4. Mix in the chard the cook and stir until the mixture is tender.
5. Toss with the pasta and sprinkle with parmesan cheese to serve.

Nutrition: Calories: 296; Fat: 9.7 g; Carbs: 44.6 g; Protein: 9.6 g

Tip: You can substitute the pasta with another any other that you like.

Harvest Pasta

Preparation Time: 35 minutes

Cooking Time: 4 minutes

Servings: 6

Ingredients:

- Kalamata olives – 1/3 cup (pitted)
- Garlic – 2 cloves (minced)
- White sugar – 1 tbsp. or more to taste
- Dried oregano – 1 tsp.
- Vegetarian burger crumbs – ¾ cup
- Diced tomatoes – 2 (14.5 oz.) cans
- Bottled roasted red peppers – 1/3 cup (chopped)
- Balsamic vinegar – 1 ½ tbsp.
- Olive oil – 2 tbsp.
- Black pepper to taste
- Penne pasta – 1 lb.

Directions:

1. In a large saucepan, stir the olives, garlic, sugar, oregano, tomatoes, red pepper, vinegar. Bring this

to simmer for about 20 to 30 minutes over medium high-heat before reducing to medium-low and let simmer until the sauce starts to thicken.

2.   In a large pot, pour lightly salted water and boil over high heat. Once the water is boiling, put in the penne pasta and leave to boil.

3.   Cook the pasta uncovered for about 11 minutes and remember to stir occasionally until the pasta is al-dente. After this drain.

4.   Once the tomato sauce is done, pour it into the blender no more than halfway full. Hold down the lid and carefully start the blender using a few pulses to get the sauce moving before leaving it o to puree. Afterwards, puree until the mixture is smooth, then return to the pot.

5.   Stir in the burger crumbles and simmer until it is hot. Then pour the finished sauce over the penne pasta to serve.

Nutrition: Calories: 392; Fat: 8.8 g; Carbs: 64.9 g; Protein: 13.4 g;

Tip: You can also use a stick blender to puree the sauce in the pot until it is smooth.

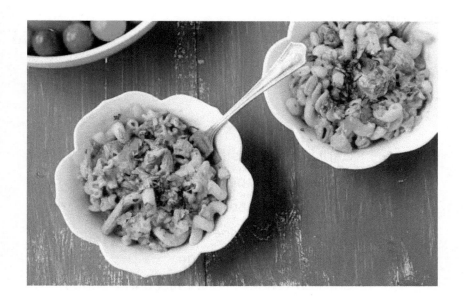

Pollo Mediterranean

Preparation Time: 25 minutes

Cooking Time: 10 minutes

Servings: 4

Ingredients:

- Olive oil – 2 tbsp.
- Garlic – 3 cloves (minced)
- Ground black pepper – ½ tsp.
- Sun-dried tomatoes packed in oi – ¼ cup (chopped and drained)
- Dry white wine – ½ cup
- Chicken tenders – 12 (sliced into strips)
- Salt – ½ tsp.
- Italian seasoning – 1 tbsp.
- Green olives – 2 tbsp. (sliced)
- Fresh parsley – 2 tbsp. (chopped)
- Sour cream – ½ cup
- Salt – ½ tsp.
- Milk – 1 cup
- Cornstarch – 1 ½ tsp.
- Water – ¼ cup

Directions:

1. In a skillet and over medium heat, heat olive oil. Place chicken and garlic in the pan. Season with pepper, Italian seasoning and ½ tsp. of salt.

2. Stir in the olives, wine, parsley, tomatoes and olives then reduce heat to a low and continue cooking until the chicken is no longer pink at the center. Remove and place chicken on a late with the sauce still in the pan. Stir into the remaining sauce ½ tsp. of sauce.

3. In a small bowl, whisk cornstarch and water together. Increase heat to the medium and whisk in the cornstarch mixture. Continue stirring until the sauce has thickened. Serve the sauce with chicken.

Nutrition:

Calories: 392; Fat: 19.7 g; Carbs: 9.2 g; Protein: 38 g;

Pasta Fagioli Soup

Preparation Time: 25 minutes

Cooking Time: 35 minutes

Servings: 6

Ingredients:

- Water – 3 cups
- Crisp cooked bacon – 8 slices (crumbled)
- Dried parsley- 1 tbsp.
- Garlic – 1 tbsp. (minced)
- Garlic powder – 1 tsp.
- Ground black pepper – ½ tsp.
- Salt- 1 ½ tsp.
- Dried basil – ½ tsp.
- Tomato sauce – 1 (8 oz.) can
- Seashell pasta – ½ lb.
- Great Northern beans – 2 (14 oz.) cans (undrained)
- Chicken broth – 2 (14.5 oz.) can
- Diced tomatoes – 1 (29 oz.) can
- Chopped spinach – 1(14 oz.) can (drained)

Directions:

1. Combine all the other ingredients apart from pasta in a large stock pot to cook and boil. Let simmer for about 40 minutes.
2. Add pasta and cook with the pot uncovered until the pasta is tender. This should take approximately 10 minutes.
3. Serve.

Nutrition: Calories: 288; Fat: 3.6 g; Carbs: 48.5 g; Protein: 15.8 mg;

Tip: You can substitute half of the canned ingredients for better nutritional outcomes.

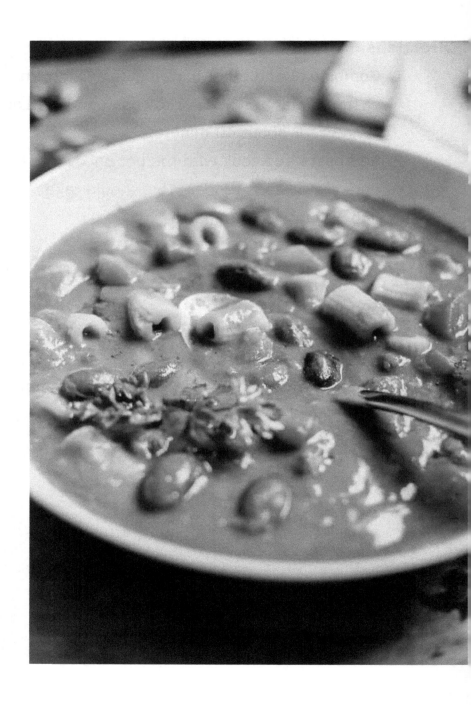

Pasta al Mediterraneo

Preparation Time: 25 minutes

Cooking Time: 15 minutes

Servings: 6

Ingredients:

- Perciatelli pasta – 1 lb.
- Pine nuts – 3 tbsp. (lightly roasted)
- Fresh parsley – 2 tbsp. (chopped)
- Lemon – 1 (juiced)
- Can tuna – 2 (5 oz.) package (drained)
- Kalamata olives – 12 (pitted and sliced)
- Garlic – 1 clove (crushed)
- Fresh basil – 4 oz. (chopped)
- Olive oil – 6 tbsp.
- Feta cheese – 2 oz. (optional)

Directions:

1. Cook pasta in a large bowl of slightly salted water until al dente. Meanwhile, mix in a large bowl, olives, garlic, basil, tuna, pine nuts, parsley and crumbled feta cheese.

101

2.   Drain the pasta. If the plan is to serve cold, then rinse the pasta with cold water until it is no longer hot. In a large bowl, place pasta together with lemon juice and olive oil. Stir into the pasta mixture, the tuna mixture.

3.   Serve hot or cold.

Nutrition: Calories: 519; Fat: 22 g; Carbs: 59.5 g; Protein: 24.2 g;

Tips: If possible, use fresh lemon juice instead of bottled ones.

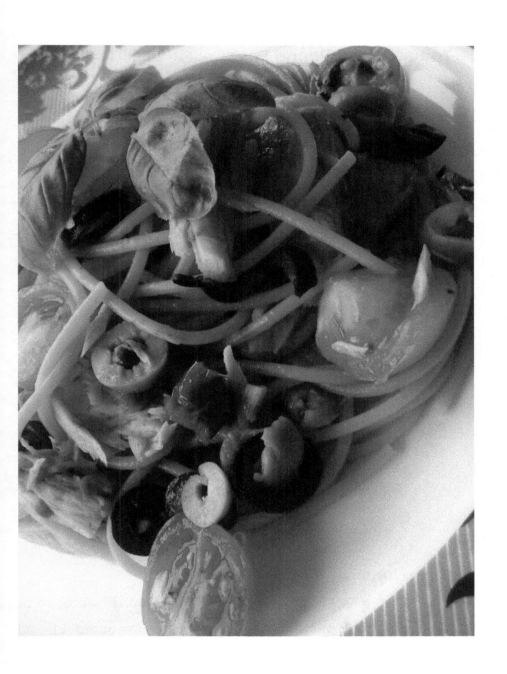

Tomato Basil Penne Pasta

Preparation Time: 45 minutes

Cooking Time: 20 minutes

Servings: 4

Ingredients:

- Basil oil – 1 tbsp.
- Garlic – 3 cloves (minced)
- Pepper jack cheese – 1 cup
- Parmesan cheese – ¼ cup (grated)
- Basil oil – 1 tbsp.
- Grape tomatoes – 1 pint (halved)
- Mozzarella cheese – 1cup (shredded)
- Fresh basil – 1 tbsp. (minced)

Directions:

1. Over high heat, bring a large pot of water to boil. Cook pasta in the boiling water for about 11 minutes until al dente, then drain.
2. In a large skillet and over medium-high heat, heat the basil and olive oil. Cook garlic in oil until

soft. Afterwards, add tomatoes, reduce the heat to a medium and leave to dimmer for 10 minutes.

3.   Stir in the mozzarella, parmesan cheese and pepper jack. When the cheese begins to melt, mix in the cooked penne pasta. Season with fresh basil.

Nutrition: Calories: 502; Fat: 24.8 g; Carbs: 47.1 g; Protein: 24.1 g;

Tip: If basil oil is unavailable, use 2 tbsp. of olive oil.

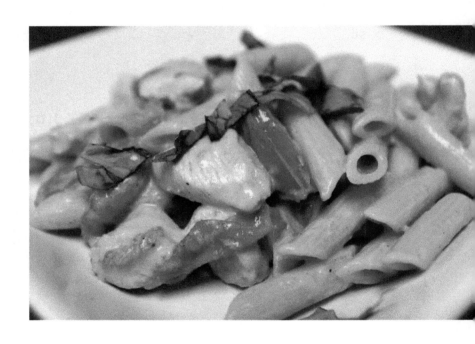

Whole Wheat Pasta Toss

Preparation Time: 25 minutes

Cooking Time: 30 minutes

Servings: 8

Ingredients:

- Olive oil – 1/3 cup
- Marinated artichoke hearts – 1 (8 oz.) jar (drained)
- Kalamata olives – ¼ cup (pitted and quartered)
- Feta cheese – ½ cup (crumbled)
- Whole wheat penne pasta – 1 (1 lb.) package
- Garlic – 4 large cloves (pressed)
- Pickled red peppers – 7 (cut into strips)
- Fresh spinach leaves – 2 cups

Directions:

1. Fill a large bowl with lightly salted water and bring to boil. Put in the penne and continue to boil. Cook the pasta uncovered, stirring occasionally for 8 minutes or until al dente, then drain.

2. In a large non-stick skillet and over medium heat, heat olive oil, the cook and stir in garlic into the hot oil for about 30 seconds until it is fragrant, for about 5 minutes. Gently fold the spinach into the mixture and stir just until slightly wilted and dark green.

3. Remove the mixture from heat and stir in the penne pasta until it is thoroughly combined; lightly toss pasta mixture in with the feta steam, cover the skillet with a lid and let the vegetables and pasta steam for about 10 minutes before serving.

Nutrition: Calories: 367; Fat :14.7 g; Carbs: 47.4 g; Protein: 12.9 g;

Quick Mediterranean Pasta

Preparation Time: 25 minutes

Cooking Time: 10 minutes

Servings: 6

Ingredients:

- Breadcrumbs – ¼ cup
- Dried basil – 1 tsp.
- Spaghetti – 8 oz.
- Dried oregano – 1 tsp.
- Olive oil – 1 tbsp.

Directions:

1. Boil slightly salted water in a large pot, put spaghetti in it and cook until al dente. Rinse and cool with water, then drain well.

2. Mix the breadcrumbs, basil, oregano and cooked pasta in a large bowl. Pour as much olive oil as you would like over the mixture and serve.

Nutrition: Calories: 178; Fat: 3.1 g; Carbs: 31.4 g; Protein: 5.5 g;

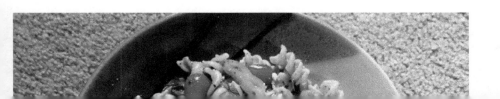

Lightning Source UK Ltd.
Milton Keynes UK
UKHW020701140521
383712UK00006B/77